$ustainable Make Millions

The *Right Way* to
Build Your Profitable,
Organic Beauty Business

Kelley Swing

The Millionaire Voice of Sustainable Beauty

Foreword

In 2017 we had the pleasure of meeting Kelley for the first time as she took on the role of being the NATULIQUE™ distributor in Texas. Looking back at the last six years, it has been an absolute privilege to watch her revolutionize the salon industry and we consider her book to be a must-read for anyone wanting to make their salon more profitable and sustainable. Especially in recent years following the pandemic, we have seen an increase in people asking for healthy, safe, organic, and sustainable products in the beauty industry. Providing these options in your salon is, therefore, absolutely key in order to stay relevant and create a profitable business.

Kelley is an expert when it comes to profitable and sustainable salons. She has worked with NATULIQUE™ for many years, and it is safe to say that a person with Kelley's passion for the salon industry is extremely rare to come across. We know Kelley to be a successful entrepreneur, businesswoman, and innovator when it comes to working with organic products. Her uncompromising approach to healthy and functional products has paved the way for increasing revenue and profit in the salons she has worked with – not to mention making the salons a healthier and more sustainable option for clients.

At NATULIQUE™, our mission is to empower hair professionals with sustainable creativity. Kelley has truly shared this mission with us and she is also extremely committed to sharing her many years of professional knowledge as a true pioneer in the industry. Consider this book a guide with specific tools and ideas for you to look inward and define how you want to run your salon in the future. If you want sustainability to be a key element on the path to increasing revenue, Kelley will share her very best advice on how to run a successful sustainable business.

In the many years to come, we look forward to seeing Kelley using her expertise to help even more people with maximizing their businesses. She is a valuable asset to the salon industry, sharing her knowledge and revolutionizing the lives of many business owners out there.

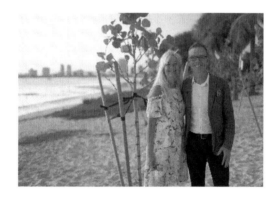

Mette   Lykkegaard   &   Stig   Bundgaard
Founders of NATULIQUE™

Foreword

When I met Kelley in 2017, her boundless devotion became immediately evident. After visiting her salon and spending time with her team, it was clear that she has an unwavering passion for creating a more sustainable future within the beauty industry. Since then, I have been fortunate to witness firsthand these dreams become a reality - an inspiring testament to Kelley's unstoppable perseverance!

Kelley has worked tirelessly to turn her salon into a million-dollar success while embodying the drive for sustainable change in the beauty industry internationally. Her majestic spirit radiates positivity and motivation - she never stops reaching greater heights! It was my privilege to mentor such fervent passion; it is inspiring how deeply she believes everyone can make a real difference when working together.

Kelley's book is an eye-opening journey through the beauty industry. After a lifetime of experience in this industry, she has created something special that every salon should read - it will change your perspective and inspire you to make sustainable changes in your business. With her insight into what truly matters in this field, listeners are guaranteed success if they follow her advice.

Kelley is a shining light in the sustainable beauty industry, and her book will show others that there can be much more to this business than meets the eye. An invaluable resource, readers are sure to benefit from its wisdom - something unfortunate generations have had to go without until now! A must-read for anyone involved or interested in the beauty world.

For those of us who have chosen this journey in life, we must constantly strive for a much more calculated and sustainable path to our consistently ever-changing and evolving destination for our children's future and the beauty industry.

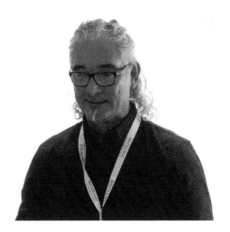

Danny Cmrelec
Managing Director NATULIQUE™ Australia
Husband, Father, Entrepreneur, Hairdresser, Educator, Brand Ambassador, Salon Owner, Mentor, Distributor, and Managing Director.

x

$ustainable Salons Make Millions: The *Right Way* to Build Your Profitable, Organic Beauty Business ©2023 Kelley Swing, The Millionaire Voice of $ustainable Beauty

ISBN: 9798388869678

Publisher:
Author Writer's Academy (AWA) Literary Agency, United States
Senior Editor: Marjah Simon
www.AWA4Life.com
Cover Design, Illustrations, and Interior Layout by Author Writer's Academy

DISCLAIMER: The content in this book is intended for educational and entertainment purposes only. This book is not intended to be a substitute for the legal, medical, psychological, accounting, or financial advice of a professional. The author and publisher are not offering professional services advice. Additionally, this book is not intended to serve as the basis for any financial or business decisions. You should seek the services of a competent professional, especially if you need expert assistance for your specific situation.

For your *Free* Download:

10 Tips on Becoming Profitably Sustainable to accompany the mastery steps in this book, while available, visit www.HeadCaseCoaching.com

Dedication

To My Daughter, **Brandy Thorpe**

You've been working in the trenches with me since Day 1. Together, we built this unique salon experience from an empty box into an amazing world of organic beauty.

Thank you for believing in my vision. I am so proud of your growth, your 'Head Case' business style as an amazing educator and leader. I could not have done this without you. I love you.

Acknowledgments

To my husband, Gregory Garlett, thank you for supporting me in every way. You fix everything in my salon so we are able to keep serving. You take care of the team that cares for our clients. Because of you, we are all happier. I love you.

My dear daughter, **Brooke Edwards**, you are the strongest person I know. You teach me how to see people's strengths and potential, and to notice the hidden gifts within them. I see you and who you are, and I am in awe of you. I love you.

To my Incredible Head Case & Innovative Beauty Team, I built the walls of the salon, but you are the heartbeat that makes it alive. Because of your talent, your love for our clients and your dedicated professionalism, we have created a truly special place. Thank you for believing in me. Thank you for trusting that Sustainable Salons are the right way to go. I love you.

To Mom and Dad, thank you for teaching me that if you work hard enough for what you want, anything is possible, no matter where you started. Dad, you showed me how leadership is an honor and how you can make a difference in people's lives. You are true testament to what it takes to be an outstanding leader. I love you.

Stig and Mette, your creation of the best products in the world, Natulique Certified Organic Beauty, brings to the industry what everyone has been wishing for. That's why I am a distributor. Thank you for your advice, coaching and leadership by example. We've been through live-changing moments together, and through it all, we became a strong family. I love you.

To Danny Cmrlec, thank you for sharing Natulique with me and opening my eyes to what's available in other countries. You are my confidant, my trainer and taught me how to handle the business side of the salon business. Your amazing support is how I learned what I can now teach - how to create and grow sustainable salons. I love you.

Table of Contents

Letter From the Author

Writing this book has been an incredible process for me. To be honest, it's been scary sharing my experiences too, but I am doing it anyway because I believe that you deserve to know what's possible and to open your eyes to the truth.

I am stepping into who I need to be to make a difference. I want to inspire sustainable change and give people the information to make the best decisions for themselves. I am speaking up about the issues that no one is being told about. Giving people hope is what means the world to me.

When I started my own journey and began to learn about the chemicals in the products I had been using for *years*, the first thing I said was, "Everyone needs to know about this!"

My new goal became to share my knowledge with as many people as possible in order to change this industry for the better. I have to prove to people that it's possible to run a sustainable, profitable, and successful business so that we can have the biggest impact on protecting our environment, the health of our stylists, and the future of this industry as a whole.

At first, I told myself I would be done when I told everyone in my salon, but then I realized I was only able to help my clients and stylists, so, I went on TV, talking about sustainability on my local network. I told myself that everyone in Keller, Texas, would surely be enough.

But after that, I sat down and thought, "No, I can't stop there. I need to reach more stylists so that they can tell their clients." I became a distributor for NATULIQUE™ - organic, cruelty-free hair products - so that I could reach even more stylists. But even after accomplishing that, I realized that I needed to do more because people are still out there buying and using products that hurt them.

I have been in this industry for as long as I can remember and am surrounded by the most incredible stylists and beauticians a girl could ask for. Even my own kids have followed me into this life.

But as a business owner, as a friend, and as a *mother*, I have a responsibility to look after my Tribe, to make sure that they know that they are loved, and they are safe with me. When I found out just how much these chemicals were hurting people, I knew it wasn't right for me to sit back and do nothing.

My stylists and my clients are my chosen family, and I want to protect my family.

That's why I'm sharing this with you now. I want to teach people what they don't know about "sustainability" in this business. I want to keep them safe and help them reach success.

In order to do that, I had to prove that my approach works. Not enough people believe that you can run a sustainable business and make money. But, after hitting a million dollars, I'm ready to share with you with 100% certainty that I've discovered something special. Something that works to support our environment that is also financially sound as a business.

I hope you enjoy reading my discoveries as I share *The Right Way to Build Your Profitable, Organic Beauty Business.*

Sustainably Yours,
Kelley Swing

Introduction

My name is Kelley Swing, and I am the voice of sustainable beauty.

The American beauty industry has been running unethically, without integrity, and down-right *dangerously* for far too long - and it's about time we do something about it.

I want to let you know that there is a way to do beauty in a sustainable way. I want to give you all the information you need to empower you to make the right decisions that are best for you and your family so that *you* can take control of your business and make strides to become the most successful version of you.

I've been doing this for six years now, raising up an extremely successful business without having to sacrifice the well-being of the people around me or my own ethics in the process.

I run a business with *people* at the very center.

You can put a building up anywhere, and you can have all the money in the world to make it look as beautiful as you want, but if you don't have the right people, your business will fail.

I'd say that I'm so lucky to have found the right people, but it's taken so much more than luck. You have to be in the right mindset and have the right reasons to be doing what you're doing so that you can create a positive culture in your salon.

The only way to do that is to work with your stylists - not just as employees, but as a whole person.

Don't get me wrong, it took us a while to get it right. I came from a corporate salon background as a district manager, running six locations. I learned a lot from that experience and brought that knowledge and some of the culture into my own business.

Most importantly, it taught me the importance of educating my team and the need for training programs. It made me seek out innovation and encourage others to change and grow.

Even though some of those practices did not generate the culture I needed for success, it gave me more credibility and confidence when I went out on my own. This background made me realize that my salon and any of my businesses had to stand for something important that could unify us in a culture that values community over competition.

So, we stand for sustainability. We created a goal and a culture that everyone feels good about. We have an ambition that gives us the capacity to help, and we love to help other stylists to do the same.

This is why I'm standing here now. This book is the start of your journey to achieve true sustainability.

But what do I mean by that? We're going to explore and give you the tools to start going for sustainability in all aspects of your salon by:

- Achieving financial sustainability - developing business acumen as a salon owner and challenging existing models of work.
- Achieving environmental sustainability - learning to take care of your planet by using products that are safe, *work* and make a profit.
- Achieving a sustainable working culture - celebrating and supporting your stylists, breaking down unhelpful stereotypes, and empowering everyone who steps through your doors.

Reading this book, I want you to believe that running your own sustainable salon is not only possible but profitable. I want to motivate you to take your first steps to success. I want to encourage you to look at the salon industry differently.

I also want to attract new people. I want to upgrade our thinking about the stereotypes around salon and beauty professionals. I want people to know that it's a really great and empowering industry - and not the stereotype of 'just for people who didn't do well in school.' I know firsthand that stylists are smart, kind, and beautiful people.

I want more people to be proud of their kids when they come into this industry because it's so much more than just 'Doing Hair.' Stylists are touching people's lives, not just their hair. They are changing lives every day, providing them with confidence and self-esteem while making art. People don't realize how much skill, effort, and time it takes to do that at an expert level. Stylists are counselors and confidants, sometimes the only person that hears them. This impacts lives. It is an honorable profession, and you can make 6-figures or more.

We have such a huge impact on people every single day. We make our clients look and *feel* beautiful and amazing. We give amazing people the confidence to show up and do the amazing things that they do all over the world.

So, let's be the change this industry needs!

SECTION I

Beauty School Dropout

Let's start where it all begins. The only way we are going to be able to change this industry is if we start addressing the stigmas and hurdles we have to face just *working* in this industry. In this section, we're going to look at:

- How we can challenge some of the negative stereotypes by seeing ourselves in a new light;
- The truth about our industry and the nuances that many aren't aware of; and
- The challenges we all face working in this industry and how we can resolve them.

Chapter 1

Challenging Stereotypes –
How Some Clients See Us

> "Everyone should be accepted
>
> for who they are."

If we really want the beauty industry to change, we have to reframe the way the world views us - because that's the only way to change the way we view ourselves.

The first time I went out to get my nails done after the COVID restrictions were lifted, those views hit me like a ton of bricks.

I was sitting in a salon between a couple of women catching up over their mani's and pedi's, so it was difficult *not* to listen to their conversation (which is never great when you're trying to relax anyway). When they got onto the topic of kids, one of them said:

"Oh, my daughter keeps getting in trouble and ditching school. She's not very smart, and she clearly doesn't want an education. So, I told her she should just go to beauty school."

I don't think I ever bit my tongue harder in my life.

First of all, she disrespected the woman in front of her who was doing her nails. Second, every person in that place could hear what she was saying, so she disrespected all of the nail technicians working around her. Thirdly, she didn't know me or my story, and she disrespected ME.

She didn't know I owned the salon across the street or that I have 20 people that work for me. She didn't know that my team is made up of some of the smartest people you will ever meet and that they work their tails off every day or that they take on every client's emotional baggage without a second thought. She didn't know that beauticians are one of the only professions that physically touch people regularly, respectfully, and allow their energy to mingle with the other person's.

Yet, in the USA, those in the beauty profession have a reputation for being stupid or that they aren't smart enough to go to college. Trade schools are just not seen to be in the same league as colleges.

The truth is beauty professionals are artists. They can see someone's head as a canvas and picture a masterpiece. They are experts in chemically creating the right color formulas for the right hair types - calculating how the hair will fall and flow, how long it will take, and how to counter any issues that may arise. They strategically put color in certain places discerning your wants in order to make it glow with color. It's pretty amazing when you think about it.

That moment in the nail salon really hit home for me. I realized it was because this woman and so many people like her would never understand that the people who work for me are very smart. But they are, first and foremost, artists.

It is a misnomer to say that a hair stylist can't make much money in this industry. I encourage you not to mistake a full-service hair salon for a quick-cut establishment because they are completely different businesses.

When you look up how much money a hair stylist could make, it will probably tell you it's around $24,000 a year, $9-$11 an hour. My stylists can actually make $100,000 a year here – even the 'juniors,' two years out of school, can make $85,000.

Despite the numbers, even some of the girls that work for me still struggle to be accepted by their own families for the work they have chosen. I have a stylist who's been on TV, worked runways, and is considered hugely successful by industry standards. Yet, some are still considered the black sheep of their family.

The two key things you need to be successful in the beauty industry are common sense and compassion. Finding someone with both qualities is a rare thing, and if you don't have them, you don't last very long. It's a unique skill set that not everyone has or can learn. So, saying that salon professionals, beauticians and artists do not do valuable work is just so damaging - especially to the well-being of these artists.

It's a ridiculous stigma that has to change.

How We See Ourselves

Not only are these stigmas completely untrue, but they are having a huge negative impact on the people coming into this industry. This misconception that 'beauty school' is a secondary option, one that parents force their kids to go to if they don't do well in school, hugely affects the morale of the students.

I have many friends who are instructors at beauty schools, and their biggest complaint right now is that a lot of the students simply don't have the drive and the commitment to be successful - let alone participate in class.

They don't want to be there. They feel like they're being forced to take a less appealing path. They're understandably upset because this line of work is associated with being less academic and, ultimately, less *successful*.

All of that, in turn, makes the instructors lose motivation. Who wants to teach a bunch of kids who don't want to be there and think your industry is a joke? It's not worth their time or talents. If the instructors don't feel like they can give their students what they need to be successful, then *they* don't feel successful.

We have to start changing this narrative. Otherwise, people will keep coming into this industry and either leave because they are convinced it's not the best place for them to be or stay and be completely unmotivated to achieve their potential.

But it's not just people starting out in the industry. Even some of my stylists and salon owners I know will joke about how they aren't good at spelling (honestly, neither am I!).

The important thing isn't about whether or not you were smart enough to go through college; it's about how much you're willing to continue your education after you finish beauty school. That is what makes a good, successful beauty professional.

As salon owners, it is our responsibility to accept our stylists where they are at and help them continue their education as they work. We have to see ourselves not just as business owners but as responsible for our stylists' engagement and growth. We have to provide them with opportunities to upskill, not just in their craft, but in other areas too.

For instance, at Head Case, we brought in a live Tony Robbins Total Results Training for all our stylists. It was really effective because it helped them to understand how and *why* they work and what it is that truly motivates them.

Everyone said they loved it. Everyone said that they learned new things about themselves that they didn't realize or made them think about habits they wanted to change.

I was speaking to someone who was especially impacted by these lessons. She realized that she'd never thought about what it is that makes her truly happy before - the thing that makes her get out of bed every morning. Tony's lessons allowed her to tap into that for the first time and work on herself and implement real change in her life.

Since then, she's been waking up early every morning and exercising for 30 minutes. She finally moved off the kitchen table to work in an office she'd made for herself. She genuinely seems happier and healthier at work, and it's just amazing to see.

Another girl told me that she finally realized who she was through those sessions. She learned her DISC personality style - found new traits she desired and what to do to learn them. It meant that we could make small changes to our teaching that made a huge impact on her development. She could gain the skills and tools that she needed to be the person she wanted to be.

But most importantly, these sessions helped bring the team together even closer. They were all coming to work from different places, different families, or financial situations. Discovering these things about ourselves meant that we had to open up to each other in ways that working the salon floor would never prompt us to.

For instance, at Head Case, we've always referred to our team as a 'family' - because, in many ways, we truly are. However, during a session, one gentleman came forward and told us he wasn't comfortable being called family. He'd had a lot of trouble and pain in his own family and didn't want to associate that with us.

If we hadn't encouraged our stylists to expand themselves, we would never have known that one of our team was suffering like this, especially over something that I would never have thought about. It allowed us to bond even further as we sat and picked out a name that felt good for *everyone*. It prompted so many people to start speaking up about ways we could make their working environment more comfortable. We came up with "Tribe" for our name.

From making tutorials more hands-on, to changing words to remove negative connotations, to even exploring more difficult topics like eating disorders, educating ourselves made us all more humble and empathetic.

This growth has allowed us at Head Case to establish a culture where everyone sees themselves as part of a *tribe* - as a group of people who are actually making a difference. They feel empowered by being a 'Head Case' because they know they're never going to leave each other behind. They love and support each other like a good family.

In order for stylists to feel that way, they have to feel comfortable. There shouldn't be any judgment if someone needs to work through something. Everyone should be accepted for who they are, regardless of what they have done or not done. If they need help, they should feel able to come to you and that you can work on it together.

The Truth About Styling and Beauty Professionals

There are a few things you have to have in order to be successful as a beauty professional. You need:

- Common sense,
- Compassion, and
- Empathy.

You have to *care* about the work you do and the people you work with, or else you will not last very long at all.

If you think about it, there are only a few professions in the world where you are expected to touch another human being. Doctors, nurses, and other medical professionals are well-respected professions and are expected to undergo a high level of education in order to interact with their patients.

Beauty professionals and hair stylists, however, are expected to touch people every single day without any of this support, education, or respect.

All day long, they coach people and listen to their problems. They take on the energy of every person they touch, which comes with a huge responsibility. The

24

truth is, it is an honor to be a stylist, to be trusted to touch people for even a moment - not just physically, but emotionally too.

Your core energy, your chakras, the position of your heart chakra, is in your chest. We all have the ability to feel whether a person is mad or sad, even if they don't tell us. This can be detected through subtle energy that radiates from an individual. As a stylist, understanding and using this innate skill is crucial for providing an exceptional experience for clients in the chair.

The area of the heart chakra is very sensitive to vibration and reflects our emotional and spiritual state. According to The Chopra Center, when our heart chakra is open, we are quick to forgive and show acceptance, kindness, and compassion towards ourselves and others.

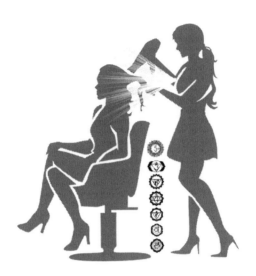

On the other hand, if this chakra is closed off, feelings such as grief, anger, and fear of betrayal may arise. Being aware of your emotional state and having an open heart allows us to provide a warm experience for clients so that we can give them our utmost care.

This also works the other way around. As stylists, your own energy is directed into the back of your client's head all day, every day. When a client is in your chair, your heart center is directly behind their head, so being cautious of the energy you send them is crucial.

If you're not in the right space, and somebody is sitting there in front of your heart, that's got to affect them. Whatever you are feeling and wherever you're at with those emotions are going to go right into your client.

I know a lot of people have a 'work persona,' a cheery version of themselves to deal with people when they themselves might be having a really lousy day. But even then, let me tell you, the client will always feel the emotion behind that mask, no matter how well you hide it.

When a client becomes uncomfortable, you will notice because their energy starts to feel off. They might be polite and tell you what you want to hear about their experience, but even if their hair is absolutely amazing, they won't come see you again.

The truth about beauty professionals is that you must be so much more than just people who "cut hair." You must be able to come to work every day as your best self or else risk making your clients uncomfortable. You have to be there for your clients and provide them with the best experience you can offer, regardless of how your own day is going.

At Head Case, we have an unofficial policy. If somebody is having an off day, we talk about it. We all know that if you're in the wrong headspace, things will start going wrong elsewhere. Sometimes it's an easy fix; sometimes, someone needs to take a walk or eat something. Other times, we need to send them home because we know that, at the end of the day, a small absence is a small price to pay for quality service.

Clients come to a beauty salon for two things:

- They want to feel better AND
- They want to look better.

It is our *job* to make sure they leave looking and feeling better and more confident.

But the other thing you need to be aware of is that you could be the only person to physically touch that person in months - maybe even years. Some people simply don't have anyone touch them except for when they go get their hair done.

It's the only other profession where you can touch someone like that. It's an intimate relationship that has the power to truly impact another person. It can change people's lives - especially those who struggle with social interaction. Stylists could be the only person to ever hear their problems, offer them a kind word, and make them feel like a human being.

There are so many stories about clients coming back to stylists to tell them they were considering suicide until they came and sat in their chair. A stylist can never

28

know what is truly going through their client's heads, but because they treat them with care and compassion, they might end up saving a life.

That is especially true when it comes to men. The CDC reports that 80% of all suicides are male[1] - which is a truly terrifying statistic. As a stylist, you have the opportunity to create an environment and a culture where people feel comfortable enough to share their feelings.

It's an honorable profession.

So, it's your responsibility to be in the best place you can be when you take on your clients because the way you feel could impact them. You never know if your client might be struggling with their mental health, experiencing depression, or even having suicidal thoughts.

That is why it is so important to understand and to know how much value your interaction has with your clients. You also need to understand the power you have to shift someone's energy with your own. The ripple effects of positive human contact could be huge.

---

[1] Centres for Disease Control and Prevention, 2020, www.cdc.gov/suicide/suicide-data-statistics.html

I think if more people understood the weight of this responsibility, they would see us as more than "just high-school dropouts." So when people talk down to beauty professionals or tell us we're a dime a dozen, I don't think they realize how much of an insult that really is.

I try my best to inspire people to look at us differently. When a nail artist is hunched over your feet all day, cleaning your feet, can you not see that as the most gracious thing a person can do? You should honor that and treat them with the respect they deserve.

SECTION 2

Chemical Warfare

I want to shed a bit of light on why green, sustainable business practice is so important in the world today. There are real and harmful consequences to the way the beauty industry operates and it simply has to change. In this chapter we will explore:

- The truth behind the chemicals we use and how they are tested;
- What other countries in the world are doing to tackle this and what *you* can do to help; and
- Why we won't stop shouting about this!

Chapter 2:

Why Should I Care?

> "To care about sustainability
>
> means to care about
>
> your own health."

When I first decided to open Head Case, there were a lot of people who told me, "Oh, that's not going to work."

Why? Well, here in Texas, big hair is everything.

Do we care how we get our big hair? No.

Starting a conversation about sustainability and the environmental impact of these beauty choices will never make you very popular. It's not that people don't care; it's that they don't know that they should.

So, I feel that it's my responsibility to teach as many people as I can.

One of the first things I like to ask people when they learn I own a salon is, "Do you know what color your stylist uses on your hair?" Nine times out of ten, they're going to say, "No, am I supposed to?"

If people don't even know the brand of product they are putting in their hair, how can you start talking to them about chemicals and animal testing? You have to meet people where they are and start educating them from there.

I had a lady come into the salon once who said to my face, "I don't care about all that stuff. I only came to your salon because it had good reviews." I was taken aback for a minute. The thing that came to mind first was that she sounded exactly like my parents. But this woman was much younger than them, and I realized then and there that I had to do something to change this kind of thinking before the next generation came along.

So I said, "That's really interesting. Let me ask you: do you really care about your health?" I reframed the conversation for her because *that* is what sustainability is about. It's about looking after ourselves, our businesses, and our planet.

If I'm talking to a salon owner, I love to tell them about how rarely my staff gets sick. It's a huge problem in our industry - and one I'll talk more about a bit later - but because of all the harsh chemicals stylists are exposed to every day, stylists are frequently off sick. As business owners, they know that when you have a lot of sick people, it can cause a lot of problems.

Running a sustainable business saves you money in so many ways. So even if you don't care about recycling (but you definitely should), you should care about sustainability because it's simply good and smart business practice.

The truth is, it's so much more than a matter of business acumen. According to the recycling company I use for all of my salon waste, Green Circle Salons, 877 pounds of beauty waste are dumped by salons every minute[2]. Every chemical we use in our salons goes straight into our water systems, tainting the water we drink and bathe in. Many products aren't only tested on animals but made using child or forced labor.

It only takes a few minutes to change your habits. So many people have a problem getting their heads around those few minutes. The tiny amount of time it takes you to put the right trash in the right bin or scoop out the product from the packaging or even remember to bring

---

[2] Green Circle Salons, www.greencirclesalons.com

along a reusable bag is so minimal. Those few minutes mean the difference between saying, 'I'm okay with this bad thing happening,' and actually making a real impact.

This is because we forget the purpose of why we're putting it into the bin in the first place. To protect our environment and the people we love.

The best way to teach sustainability is to focus on the *why* behind it before we can do the rest of the steps. That is so much easier than trying to enforce all these rules on people. Once people start doing it, everyone loves it, and when people get excited about it, they will tell other people about it.

I have a stylist who recently went to a barber show, but because she was so used to recycling absolutely everything when she works with us at Head Case, she asked the guys there where she should put the swept-up hair. She said they looked at her like she was insane!

When things like this become common practice in your salon, it just becomes a habit. You don't think about how many extra minutes you're spending doing it - and most of the time, it doesn't take any longer anyway!

So many of my clients tell me that they never really recycled until they started coming to our salon. Now, their whole family is doing it. If you think about how many people's lives you can touch with just a little bit of education, we can make real change.

The Dark Side of Beauty

I never had any allergies or health problems until I started working in a salon. I started in the industry by managing and was never behind the chair. Those first few years, working with 25 stylists and inhaling ammonia all day long made me sick all the time. I'm not even a stylist, yet I started getting respiratory problems, sinus infections and my hair even started falling out.
I didn't know what was happening to me.

I spent some time away from the beauty industry after I moved to California to work in a hospital. I worked in the radiology department where we did hundreds of mammograms, CAT scans and MRIs, and I started to notice a pattern with some of the people coming in. What caught my attention was the number of 20-somethings coming in.

At first, I was always telling them not to worry. When you're in your 20s, lumps, and bumps are usually benign, and we usually only do scans as a precaution. But what started to happen was more and more, we would take a look at the first scans and ask them to come back in for more testing. Then see them again a few months later for a CAT scan. Before I knew it, these girls were getting cancer treatments.

At the time, I had two daughters, and it was just absolutely terrifying to me. I kept thinking, "I wonder what this is? How can I make sure they don't end up coming to see me at work?"

It wasn't until I went grocery shopping one day that it caught my eye. It was an 'organic' hair salon, and I remember thinking, "Yeah, sure, like that will ever work."

I thought there was no way to get a decent hair color with natural ingredients, but I was curious, so I spoke to the woman. She told me about all the misconceptions about organic products and how damaging a lot of the chemicals in mainstream products were.

That conversation sent my brain into overdrive. Suddenly, so many of my health issues started to make sense. It completely opened my eyes. When I left, I knew that even though I didn't have the answers, I had the questions, and I was going to find out.

I started studying and researching, and examining all the products in my house.

And oh my God!

What I found was shocking. You see, the hair follicles on your scalp are three times larger than the ones on your arm.

Now, think about how much product your scalp takes in - every bit of bleach, every drop of hair color, every ounce of relaxer. Think about what organ is directly under your scalp.

When you think about how many hairs there are per follicle in African-American hair, and the relaxers and straightening treatments, there's no wonder why there's such a high percentage of people getting cancer. All those chemicals have direct access to our bloodstreams and it makes us sick.

And we all sit there, every four-six weeks, letting this stuff rot on our heads. I've done it; I've done it to my daughter's hair without even thinking about it.

When I thought back to all those girls who came in for mammograms at the hospital - I realized *this* might be why they were all getting sick. Stylists work with permanent hair dye and chemical hair straightening products day in and day out. It gets on their hands and on their skin and it's literally giving them breast cancers[3]. In a study that came out in 2019, they found there is, "a higher breast cancer risk associated with hair dye use, and the effect is stronger in African American women, particularly those who are frequent users"[4].

I have one client who had cancer three different times and was told by her doctor is was from being a hair stylist and she needed to stop doing hair. I have another who had bladder cancer who was also told to stop doing hair because their cancer was chemically induced from being a hair stylist.

I started researching everything I could find and telling everyone that I knew that something was very wrong. I checked all the products in my bathroom and called my mom and my girls, and told them to just get rid of everything.
As soon as those products were out of my life, I immediately started to notice my respiratory issues fading. I started buying organic wherever possible, and I just kept getting better and better.

---

[3] International Journal of Cancer, 2019, www.onlinelibrary.wiley.com/doi/10.1002/ijc.32738
[4] National Institutes of Health, 2019
https://www.nih.gov/news-events/news-releases/permanent-hair-dye-straighteners-may-increase-breast-cancer-risk

So when I went back to the beauty industry and opened up my own salon, I knew I wanted to do things right. I wanted to give everyone the information they needed to empower themselves to make those informed choices.

But even that had its hurdles.

For about a year, I started with a company that claimed their products that were natural and organic. I took what they were saying at face value when I should have questioned it much sooner than I did.

When we used their colors, the results were never consistent. After a while, I started researching and using other brands to try and figure out why the results were so inconsistent and find a brand that I could trust.

I discovered that if a manufacturer has one item in their line that is organic, natural or ammonia free, some of them claim the entire line as being organic or natural!

That's like saying water is pure water, even though you've got a drop of cyanide in it.

When I looked at this 'organic' product that I'd been using all year, this was exactly the case. I knew that I would not be able to represent this brand any longer because I had made promises to give our clients the cleanest and safest products I could find. I had failed.

US Laws Compared to EU Laws

In the US, companies are allowed to sell you an entire bottle of toxic chemicals as 'organic' as long as it contains a small amount of something organic.

Because of this, I would personally never trust a product that was made in the US. When I looked at the 'organic' product I was talking about in the last chapter, I had been fooled into thinking it was made in Australia. But when I asked my Australian friends about it, they told me to actually go look at the bottle. There, in the small print, it said, 'Made in the USA.'

When you look at the EU and the UK, they have so many stringent laws about which chemicals are even allowed in the country. All of their products are produced according to the strictest cosmetic laws and follow the EU Cosmetics Directive's ban on 1,328 chemicals from cosmetics that are known to cause cancer, genetic mutation, harm, or birth defects[5].

---

[5] European Commission, Legislation, www.single-market-economy.ec.europa.eu/sectors/cosmetics/legislation_en

In the US, we only have a ban on 11 of them[6]. This list does not include ammonia.

Another example of this would be the product lines in Australia compared to the US. If you buy a box of products in Australia, for example, the box will come with warning labels. Black labels that say clearly: these products contain chemicals that are harmful to your health. When you order those same products here in the US, they have absolutely nothing on them about health warnings because they are not regulated by the FDA or USDA.

There is simply very little regulation of hair care products in the US. It means that every day we are using products that the global market has deemed unsafe for use.

This might seem extreme, but I was 19 years old when I first got my cancer diagnosis. It taught me that it's important to always ask questions and seek second opinions. That experience also showed me how powerful your gut feeling is when making decisions about personal health matters.

---

[6] FDA, as of 2022, www.fda.gov/cosmetics/cosmetics-laws-regulations/prohibited-restricted-ingredients-cosmetics

Removing these products from my life gave me near-instant relief from my ongoing respiratory issues. I felt happier, healthier, and I could literally breathe *easier* when I wasn't using them every day. Not only that, but when I implemented this same rule in my salon, my stylists stopped getting sick to the same degree.

When I talk about how sustainability *is* profitable, this is what I mean right here. But this goes so much *much* deeper than just saving money by maintaining a reliable service. **This is about people's lives.**

If you want to go even deeper into examining your products, I can recommend you look out for a few key ingredients that are being researched as carcinogenic - which means that the ingredient causes cancer and helps cancer grow.[7]

The chemicals that you should be avoiding in haircolor are:

- PPD (P-phenylenediamine)
- PTD (toluene-2,5-diamine)
- Hydrogen Peroxide
- Ammonia

---

[7] NATULIQUE, www.natulique.com/safe-hair-colors-after-cancer/

- Parabens
- Resorcinol
- Lead Acetate
- DMDM Hydantoin

My family has been affected by this, my work family has been affected by this and there is a better way.

Chapter 3:

Safe Waste

"There is still
so much work
to be done."

When I talk about ethical and environmental sustainability in salons, I mean that everything you do should be for the betterment of the planet. Ensuring that everything you do, every product you use, is certified organic, natural, and sustainable so that you aren't causing any harm to yourselves, your clients, or to the environment and water supplies.

In my opinion, the beauty industry is causing more damage to the world than any other profession.

When you have a salon on every corner using products containing ammonia or other harsh chemicals, and all these horrible chemicals are getting washed down your drain, where do you think they end up? They end up in your local water system.

Did you know that hair lets off methane gas when disposed of improperly? A recent study showed that "When natural hair inside plastic bags sits in a landfill, it can produce methane, a powerful greenhouse gas. There are many possible uses for human hair waste, but they require hair to be disposed of in a responsible way in order to mitigate any environmental risks."[8]

So now we have to look at the landfill statistics and how we combat that. Here are a few ways in which we at Head Case are challenging these situations. We recycle hair through an organization that repurposes the hair into hair booms, hair-stuffed nets which are used to soak up oil spills in the ocean. They have also started repurposing hair into plastic tubes for playgrounds. We never throw our hair foils in the waste but recycle them instead. Everything we use in the salon is cruelty-free so that no animal, child, or slave is affected in the production of the products we use. Many of our products are packaged with ocean-friendly recycled plastics and created with certified organically farmed ingredients.

Here are some other ways you could actively create a more sustainable business strategy in your salon.

---

[8] Is Hair Biodegradable or Does it Harm the Environment?', by Arebella Ruiz, *The Round Up*.

1. **Create a recycling program** - Look at where your waste is currently going and see if you can find ways to make improvements. Everything can be recycled; it might just take a little more research to find companies in your area that will do it. When switching over, encourage clients with old shampoo or conditioner bottles to bring them in for recycling. This would give them the incentive to purchase these items sooner and provide an opportunity for environmentalism.

2. **Focus on community impact** - Find a way to make an impact that aligns with your company values but also evokes change in your local community. For instance, if you partner with companies that distribute cruelty-free products, consider supporting your local humane society with a yearly dog and cat food drive.

3. **Go paperless** - Buy reusable drinkware and cutlery instead of disposable ones. Email client receipts instead of printing, and build your email list simultaneously. Install a hand dryer in the restroom instead of paper towels. Reuse old product containers as decorations and plant flowers in them.

4. **Make the switch to sustainable products -** Your products should resonate with the values you hold. When looking for sustainable brands to represent your business, I advise getting clarity on what their core beliefs and principles are — not only to support them but to also ensure they align seamlessly with your company's purpose as well.

5. **Get your clients involved** - Inspiring sustainable change is a great way to inspire others and help make your community better.

These are some quick changes you need to make to get you started on the road to sustainability. By helping to preserve the planet, you are telling people who you are and what you represent.

Empowering Yourself With The Truth

When you start talking to people about sustainability in the salon industry, the first thing they are going to say is that it doesn't work. Even if they do believe it's possible, the second thing they're going to say is that it costs too much.

But the truth is, the beauty industry is designed to waste your money. It will purposefully sell you products that are lower quality, so you have to buy more. It will dress up the same product in different packaging, so you think you're getting a product that is best for your hair type and color. It will put chemicals on your head that aren't necessary for even cleaning your hair - just because we, as a consumer, have learned to associate that 'soft, silky, straight out the shower' feeling with cleanliness. Let me tell you right now, it's just coating your hair in silicones.

Educating yourself and empowering yourself with the truth is the only way to challenge this. Do your homework and read the product details. When I was using those 'Australian' products, I believed the product was organic purely based on what I was told instead of doing my own research. Because I trusted them, I was contributing to this problem.

If you're beginning your journey to sustainable, healthy, and organic hair, my best advice would be to look at the product you're using and see if it says 'made in the USA' anywhere on the bottle. If it does, I would seriously suggest throwing it away.

Until the USA decides to ban carcinogenic chemicals from our products, I wouldn't trust it. If you find a small company that has consciously decided to give you clean products, I would ask you to visit their warehouse to see for yourself. If they are pure, then they should welcome the visit.

As a salon owner, ask your product suppliers for a Material Safety Data Sheet or 'SDS' as they are now called - this is something that they are required, by European law, to have for all their products. Many US suppliers won't give this out willingly or just don't have one, especially since US law does not require this. In the US, products such as drugs, cosmetics, food or alcoholic beverages, wood or wood products, tobacco or tobacco products, or articles (finished goods) are exempt from the SDS portion of the hazard communication standard.⁹

But you can still ask for it.

---

⁹Code of Federal Regulations, 29CFR1910. 1200(b)(6)(viii)

When we asked our 'organic, Australian-made' product supplier for the SDS, it showed that there was 4-11% ammonia in a product that was labeled as 'ammonia free.'

For those who don't know what ammonia is or does, it's a toxic, corrosive chemical that (in high enough quantities) can cause respiratory failure, cancers, and even death. Now, imagine you're a stylist working with these products every day, every week for months on end, inhaling these chemicals. I've said it before, but now you see why so many stylists get sick.

But it's not just the stylists; it's the clients too.

So what is the solution?

When we got the SDS sheet on those products, I honestly had no idea where to even begin. So, if you're feeling overwhelmed by any of this information, please know that it's not your fault. Unfortunately, we live in a country that does not have effective chemical regulations. There isn't enough *education* for people to learn about the long-term effects of these chemicals.

Products You Believe In

In order for you to sell products and ask your stylists to sell them, you must genuinely believe in them. No one wants to sell or be sold something they don't need. So your stylists have to be able to trust their products, identify a problem the client has and prescribe them something to fix it.

I'm a distributor for the product line NATULIQUE™. The way we work is that in order for you to take a product from me and sell it yourself, I have to train you on how to use it properly. It's a one-on-one process - which means that every seller is essentially an expert and can give the client the best possible experience when purchasing.

Not only that, but everything about the product is good for you, your wallet, and the environment:

Everything they create, they create using wind power and green energy;

They only ever use ingredients that are organically farmed;

Every product they make must be beneficial for the hair and the scalp.

Their packaging is made from recycled materials to create bottles that can be recycled again after use; and

Nothing they create is tested on animals and is completely cruelty-free.

But this is an industry that is full of competition. A lot of the bigger companies have stopped using distributors because it's cheaper to sell online or pay a bunch of influencers to market your product. There's no personal contact, no camaraderie, and no expert opinion to help guide a client to the right product to suit their needs.

Every single product line you can find on Amazon claims to be recommended by a salon professional.

The truth is that people actually *want* a product to be recommended by a hairstylist. It sure beats standing in a store scanning hundreds of different products, all claiming to do the same thing.

What I do love about NATULIQUE™ is that they've made this process so much simpler. Clients can order online from your salon, but they don't sell mass retail in stores or on their website. That means if another salon wants to use the products, they have to come through us, the distributors.

It's a boutique line, and we're selling it with a guarantee that the product isn't going to change. I've found through my experience working in this industry that companies often start with good intentions and all these promises that their product line will always deliver on quality. However, after a while, you start to notice that the product isn't working the same way it used to. Six months later, the company will come out and say, "Oh, by the way, we changed the formula."

You can see this especially when large companies take over other brands. When industry giants take over other smaller companies, they frequently sign a contract with that company that states they won't change the formula for their products for a certain number of years. But, as soon as that time period expires, there is nothing stopping them from doing exactly that. This is common practice in the beauty industry and others.

I have a client who used to be a brand ambassador and educator for a beauty company for years. Her courses were three days long and in person, and everyone had to go through that course in order to learn about the company and its products.

When this company was bought out by a larger one, everything changed. According to my client, as soon as the 'no changes' contract ended and the new company took over completely, they terminated her position and eliminated that entire training culture. My friend said that the courses she ran were turned into an hour-long video and that, in her opinion, the products that are coming out are definitely not the same quality anymore.

It's something to be aware of - especially as more and more brands start to push their 'sustainable' product lines. As environmental causes become much more prevalent in the public eye, we are starting to see these big brands try to respond to this market.

What is actually happening is that they might introduce a new "natural" product line, which is not the same as "certified organic," but they will continue to create their core products that are made with ingredients that were outdated 30 years ago. Those are still full of chemicals.

So yes, the industry has taken a shift in the right direction, but there is still so much work to be done, and there are still going to be products out there that will try and sell you false information. Just because the packaging is green or says natural or organic doesn't mean it's good for you.

This is why it's so important to find a brand you can trust. NATULIQUE™ has been creating salon professional products for over 20 years. They know what they're talking about and are doing everything they can to decrease their environmental impact even further.

Using The Power of the Dollar
by Buying Organically

As I've said before, when you look at the huge organizations in the beauty industry, you'll notice that they will have thousands of different products, often under the same brand. What they don't tell you is how often these products contain exactly the same chemical compound. The only difference is the packaging.

These companies know that consumers want a *personal* experience when we shop and they will do anything to make us think that their products are tailored to you specifically. The reality is, they aren't. They use these marketing tactics to lure you in and you often pay twice as much as its counterpart with less glamorous packaging.

When we buy certified organic products - products that are transparent about their contents - we are telling these corporations what it is that we actually value: authenticity.

If you buy NATULIQUE™, you know that not only are all the products certified organic and sustainable, several of them are made from biomass products. This means all are made from leftover wheat and corn chaff, all the stuff that usually gets burned after harvesting. Instead, they take it and recycle it and use it to replace harmful gas in aerosol sprays.

When you buy something by NATULIQUE™, it's all product. You can spray a tiny little bit of mousse on your hand, and it might only look like a small drop - but as soon as you rub it in, it becomes a lotion. You can cover all your hair with just one drop, which means some of the products can last anywhere between four to six months.

Let's talk color. What if you had a color line that worked 100% of the time and lasted longer? As a salon owner, consistency is key to success. If you can count on your color to deliver every time, you save money on unnecessary redos and client complaints. Priceless.

We measure everything we use at Head Case to reduce waste. We found that from just one tube, you can get three or more root touchup color applications. If you think about how much you pay for an average tube of color vs. how many applications you get, it's really a no-brainer.

NATULIQUE™ styling products last at least twice as long as competitor brands. Some last up to 5 times longer, which could mean significant savings for your clients. Let's figure out the math:

- If you bought a product for $36 every month for 12 months, that is $432 per year.
- If you bought a product that would last two times longer, your cost would be $216.
- If you bought a product that would last three times longer, your cost is $108 and a savings of $324.

How much would you save on your salon's back-bar if the products lasted twice as long?

If you have ten stylists using an $18 product and you replace it monthly, that is $2160 for the year. Suppose you replace this product half as many times, which is $1080. If you replace this product only three times, your cost is $540, with a savings of $1650 on just one product.

But let's go even further. What if you had that miracle styling product that worked on all hair types? Wouldn't you need fewer back-bar items to buy, store, and replace? How much cost savings would this be?

Switching out your current products for NATULIQUE™ would provide your clients with affordable, long-lasting products. You would make significant savings on your stylist's back-bar. You would be making a huge step towards becoming a sustainable business that actually cares about the well-being of its people and our planet. You could do all that just by using the NATULIQUE™ product line. Yes, I do love my NATULIQUE™!

SECTION 3

The System Is Broken

I do not believe that the beauty industry can continue the way that it is. Especially not successfully. In this section, I want to shed light on the systems in place that stop us from making any positive progress and how you can challenge them. We'll be looking at:

- The systems that are actively working against us to devalue our skills;
- How taking advantage of people and burning bridges will get you nowhere in the long run; and
- The power of a good business education.

Chapter 4

Stop Devaluing Our Industry

"People come into your life
for a season or a reason."

We've already talked about how difficult it can be to be taken seriously as a hairstylist. But here in the US, it's not just public opinion that we are fighting against.

Currently, in order to be a stylist here, you have to obtain a license. That means there is a degree of training that is mandatory for everyone who handles hair.

As I've said before, this is so important because being a stylist comes with the responsibility of touching another human being. It needs to be taken very seriously, and it's not something that many people are even prepared for. There is so much value in their interactions with clients who are potentially lonely or vulnerable.

At Head Case, I'm constantly investing in my people to help them continue their education. I also invest in myself, so I can run a better business. When you invest in yourself, you're going to have more pride in your job, and you're going to care about what you're doing. You're going to attract more people that feel the same.

However, in 2019, there was a movement in Texas to take this licensing away. That is absolutely insane to me. That would have meant that anybody could open up a salon and start working without going through the process of educating themselves. Texas HB 1705 proposed to eliminate cosmetology licensing but was later modified to conduct a study to "...determine what improvements, if any, can be made to remove obstacles to employment and reward hard work, while continuing focus on keeping Texans safe."[10] The sponsor of the bill made that determination after discussions with constituents and industry professionals.

Removing the licensing requirement, would have devalued the professional hair stylist who has taken the time to go to school and get an education and then is put in the same position as someone else who did none of that work.

---

[10] www.kxxv.com/hometown/texas/texas-lawmaker-house-bill-1705-will-no-longer-abolish-cosmetology-license-requirement

We fought against it here in Texas and I know there are other states that are already going through the process of trying to implement the idea of removing the requirement for cosmetology licensing. Nebraska LB 189 amends the Cosmetology, Electrology, Esthetics, Nail Technology, and Body Art Practice Act in the Nebraska code, "to provide for an exemption for natural hairstyling,"[11] which removes the need for a cosmetology license to practice 'hairstyling'.

If you would like to find out more and have your say, Change.org has a petition to sign if you want to help in the fight to keep licensing in Nebraska.

It's all a way for business owners to save money by not having to recruit from the small pool of people who have actually successfully got their licenses. They can hire anyone they like and pay them $9 an hour to do it. They don't even have to care or invest in their future at all.

If they take that license and educational requirement away, then not only are we not going to have anyone good in our salons, but the clients will suffer.

---

[11] LB189, Nebraska Legislature, 2023

Would you want someone without a license and training to put chemicals on your head? Would you trust someone without a license and training to touch your feet or cut your hair? This is a skilled job that has a huge responsibility for the well-being of its clients.

One of the things people don't think about is sanitation. When you get your license, you need to prove that you are capable of managing a high level of sanitation for your clients. There is a huge difference between practicing sanitation physically every day and doing a session online. Do you know how many people we see in a week and the level of sanitation that is necessary for our client's safety, not to mention our own? Do you know how many times someone sat in that chair or put their head in that bowl?

These are just some of the health practices which are covered under education and training for licensing and maintaining the license. Practices that are vital for keeping a safe and sanitized working environment for both stylist and client.

In my opinion, instead of rallying for non-licenced stylists, we should be advocating for the commission salon. It is a sustainable business model that works to develop stylists who are looking to start their journey in the industry for stability, education, growth opportunities, consistency, support and camaraderie.

I want to take a moment to tell you what the key differences are between a commision salon and your average 1099, booth rental salon.

At Head Case, being a commission salon means that I pay all my stylists a wage. I pay their taxes, I give them a commission on what they do. I also train them and provide all their products. They work with Head Case clients as an employee, as a unit. There is structure that is key to developing a stylists education and understanding of the standards needed to be successful in the industry. For example, we have a dress code - which means from the very beginning, you can't show up in your pajamas.

But booth rental places work differently. As a stylist, they're hiring their chair from someone else. This means they are completely on their own when it comes to running their business. It's also against the law for a 1099 salon owner to treat their stylists as employees but a lot of places still do this as a way to 'save money'.

There simply isn't that same level of structure as in a commission salon and stylists can pretty much do what they want. If you combine this with unlicensed stylists, not only are you going to have a completely unmotivated and broken system but the value of the trained professional will plummet.

Beauty School

I've said it before, but the issues with the beauty industry as an institution start with its foundation: beauty school.

We have young students going to beauty school for all the wrong reasons: their parents make them do it, they think it's the only alternative if they don't do well in high school, or it could even be that they thought it sounded more interesting than shop.

We know already that if we don't challenge the discourse about stylists and beauticians, this situation is only going to get worse. Teachers will become mentally spent trying to work with students who don't care. It will become a less desirable job, and you'll stop getting quality instructors teaching these kids.

This brings me to the biggest issue I see with beauty schools: the poor curriculum. People are leaving school without realistic expectations of the industry, no business acumen, and how to screw over established salons by stealing their clients.

When I recently asked a stylist a year after they had finished beauty school how many of their graduating class are still in the industry, they told me they didn't know of anyone. Not only is that a waste of $30,000, but it's also a waste of everybody's time, even though you don't get much of an education anymore. Since COVID, beauty schools in Texas have dropped 500 hours of practical education.[12]

One of the problems is that the curriculum sells students on the idea that becoming a beauty professional is to 'Be Your Own Boss.'

Sure, it sounds amazing when you're told that you can make your own schedule or bring your kids to work and live your life on your own terms. But they never tell them how to actually do it.

The realities of getting to that point in your career are so much more complicated than graduating and immediately setting up shop. You don't go from standing by a chair one day to swimming in money the next, especially if no one has ever taught you how to schedule yourself and you only turn up to work when you feel like it.

---

[12] Texas Department of Licensing and Regulations, 2021, www.tdlr.texas.gov/cosmet/cosmetfaq.htm

You have to educate them on how to run a *business*. But even then, it's not for everyone. It takes a lot of work, and you need to be in the right headspace and have enough resilience to see it through.

It's one of my biggest irritations when a client asks a stylist, "When are you going to get your own salon?" As if a stylist can only be *successful* if they are in their own booth other than working at a reputable salon. People have this huge misconception about what success in the beauty industry looks like. They don't ever consider that stylists might love what they're doing exactly where they are and how they are doing it.

Yet, beauty schools continue to teach students that's exactly what they need to do. They don't teach them how to do their marketing or how to register their business properly, or even build their own website. They seem to teach them to go into an established salon, build a clientele, and then leave, taking as many people as they can with them.

When that happens, it doesn't seem to matter whether they've signed a non-compete agreement. Some people will create lies and other negativity about the salon they are leaving so they can justify doing it.

This practice is completely ruining commission salons. Every time this happens, they take several thousand dollars of client income a week. All the marketing the salon owner has spent on that person, all the products and training they provide them with, and all taxes they've paid all go down the drain. It's stealing, but no one looks at it that way. It generates such a terrible, hurtful culture in this industry, and there are so many better ways to thrive without stabbing people in the back. Many commission salons have closed down because of this reason.

The bottom line is this: in order to be successful as an independent stylist, you have to have a business education and ethically start your business by building it yourself. If you have the drive, stamina, and financial backing to do so, I support you 100%. I have some very successful and amazing independent stylists as my clients today.

If you're coming straight out of beauty school, your first move should be to find a commission salon that is committed to furthering your education and a place to call your forever home.

You could even find an apprenticeship program like the one we created at Head Case. It's a six-month to two-year program, depending on your experience, where you would be trained to thrive in the beauty industry.

During that time, you would shadow my stylists and work with my team and educators. You would work on models every week until your skills grow and you're able to produce exceptional work. Then you would have the opportunity to get on the floor and become a commissioned stylist with us. All of that happens while you are being paid for your apprenticeship work.

Feel like applying?

Call us on 682-593-7425

1200 Keller Parkway, Suite 400, Keller, Texas 76248

Just give us a call and stop by the salon when you can. Let us prove to you that by supporting each other and surrounding yourself with people that encourage you to grow, you can become the stylist you're meant to be.

Booth Renting

People come into your life for a season or a reason.

When you look at other countries like Australia, they have it absolutely right. They actively debate and implement laws to support and protect stylists - especially those coming straight out of beauty school.

Their model is fairly simple. After beauty school, a stylist has to do a two-year apprenticeship in a salon where they are paid a fair working wage by the salon owner. When those two years are up, they can choose to stay at the salon or move on to another salon.

During those two years, everyone works together like a unit. The new stylist is learning from the community around them and getting a deeper understanding of how the business works. The salon owner has a reliable stylist who they want to nurture because it's in their best interest to keep them working there as long as possible. I recently had an update that the booth rental model is now becoming more prevalent after COVID due to people offering hair services at home during the shut downs. Many salon owners are concerned about where the industry is now going due these changes.

However, when you look at the booth rental model we have here in the US, the culture is just so much more competitive.

This might be an unpopular opinion, but it needs to be said: The Booth Renting System is a challenging model, which has increased in recent years. It's something that beauty schools cling to as a way of promoting their classes and selling their school. They're making promises that are not true.

What the schools are actually doing is pushing students onto the Booth Renting conveyor belt - which is a fundamentally broken system - without actually giving them any of the tools they need to market or build a business. They teach them how to take a test, and then that's it. They're out on their own, and the only path they've been taught is booth rental.

If you're reading this and wondering what I'm talking about, booth renting is when you approach an established salon and pay to use a chair. You are working as an 'independent' stylist, with access to the clients and sometimes the benefit of the front desk to manage appointments. In theory, it is a way for stylists to earn more money by becoming a business owner.

But, despite what the beauty schools tell them, they're not salon owners.

Yes, they are in charge of their work, manage their rent and finances, and show up when they want. But because they don't have the support network of the salon, many are constantly making bad decisions.

The only person they're accountable to is themselves, so it doesn't matter if they show up in their sweatpants or decide not to show up at all. They can try and charge you three times more than local competitors without thinking too hard about it because they don't have the business acumen to know how to do that research.

So for salon owners, you're getting unreliable, unchecked, and overpriced stylists - but even worse, if you do take these stylists under your wing, there is the risk that they might do something to ruin your reputation. Booth renting is often also the only way for some stylists who have been let go from other salons to continue their trade.

Because of the booth renting system, it is too easy for stylists to go behind your back and leave you by renting a new booth somewhere else. Frequently, they recruit your other booth renters and attempt to take your clients with them. At Head Case, I've always done my best to support *all* of my stylists. I educate them, train them, let them take on our clients, and build them up so that they can grow in the industry.

So many hairstylists want to own their own salon, but that's simply not possible for every single artist. They can be the smartest, most creative person, but if they do not have that analytical, business part of the brain, they will never be successful. They simply don't have the management or leadership skills to run a salon. Too often, stylists are mistreated simply because the owner just doesn't know any better.

How is teaching students to go behind established salon owners' backs a sustainable practice? How is it ethical if the people leaving have to lie to justify the fact they're leaving, like telling people that something's wrong with the salon or they're going to own their own place? How is it sustainable to poach clients, taking contact information on the fly, so they can try to start their business?

This is how it works. Say a new stylist comes in for six months, learns what they think are all the tricks of the trade, and then decides they can do it better themselves. They recruit a few friends who also work at the salon to join them because they can't afford the whole rent of a new place on their own. They all burn their bridges with the former salon owner so that they can make their escape without anyone looking too closely at their contract. It's highly unethical, and even if they're under a non-compete contract, they'll try to do it anyway because that's what they're told to do in beauty school or from friends in the industry.

When that happens, it hurts every person involved.

It hurts the clients, who are messed around, have their appointments canceled, and no longer trust their salon or stylist;

It hurts the salon itself, which has to take the hit of losing multiple stylists and the backlash of whatever reason they claimed to be leaving; and

It hurts the stylists because they simply do not have the business skills to establish themselves on their own and will often fail because of this.

I'll never forget the last time this happened to me. It was right before Christmas, and I had never felt so defeated. I've had people leave before and take clientele when I thought that they would never do so. Every time I'm really surprised and hurt.

That time, I had three people leave two weeks before Christmas. They all recruited each other, talking bad about the business because they had to justify their behavior. Then they posted on social media how terrible we were.

They walked right out the door in front of a salon full of people!

I remember looking at my front desk leader, who's been with me right from the start, and we both just started crying.

Ashley has had to call clients so many times and say, "I'm so sorry. Your stylist left. Can we reschedule you?" She's lost so many friends, people she'd grown close to, and then they abruptly left. I've lost count of how many times my daughter has told me, "I don't want to do this anymore." It just kept happening and happening.

My first reaction to the three that left at Christmas was to serve them all Cease and Desist (orders from the court requiring them to halt their business activities). They had all broken contracts, recruiting clients and stylists.

But when I actually sat down and thought about what I wanted, I thought, what's the path of least resistance? I can go to court and sue every one of these girls, knowing full well that they are making absolutely nothing. I could pay for a much better lawyer than they could and cause a lot of animosity and grief.

Or I could not. I could decide that I didn't need them and just keep going. I hear today only one is still working in the industry.

So that's what we did, and we finally figured it out. Even after we went through all those hardships, we came out of it with an amazing team.

This is why there are fewer and fewer commission salons left. Established salons don't want to put up with the hassle anymore, so they close down.

So many times, I have thought that I'm just going to quit. We're not going to get out of this hole, and we should just close. But then, guess what? Each time, we got out of the hole.

Then I realized that it was not about me; it was about something else. It's about where people are in their life and where they work with you. People come into your life for a season or a reason.

I was talking to one of my coaching clients who was going through this exact same thing. She'd had a few people walk out and was just stuck in that horrible headspace of "I'm just going to quit." She literally tried to sell me her salon!

But because I've been through it all, because I *know* how it feels, I was able to relate to her on a much deeper level. I was able to look her in the eye and say, "Listen, you're going to be fine. You're going to get through this." I could say that because I know from my own experience that if you stick at it and learn from your lowest moments, you're on track to get to a place where you're doing even better than you've ever done before.

I know it's hard, and I know that it feels like a really rough time. It's hard being a business owner anyway, but in this industry, where you're asked to give so much of yourself and get so close to people who may walk away at some point, it can be devastating. I have learned to stop talking about them, not to give them another thought, and to turn my focus on my incredible and loyal employees.

Coming out the other side means putting your energy into building your company instead of getting caught up in your hardships. I've always believed in karma, so if you just put one foot in front of the other, do the right thing, and follow the rules, you'll at least be able to sleep at night.

It's so sad that people come into our lives and miss the opportunity they had, but that's not your problem. Your problem is figuring out how you move forward without anyone else getting hurt along the way.

At my salon, we have learned from this. We have now created a culture where we are educating all of our stylists about the pros and cons of working a booth and why commission salons work the way they do. And guess what? When people are educated about the risks they are taking, and you create a good and open culture about it, people don't want to leave.

But if my stylists do decide to go, it's great if they do so on good terms. It's important to me that the stylists that work for me know that they can call me up in six months' time and say, "Hey, it didn't work out. Can I come back?" I will even support them if they leave on good terms and do it ethically, which I have for a few who are clients of my distribution company.

In this industry, it's important to never burn a bridge if you don't have to. By promoting open and honest conversation with your stylists, not only are you creating a salon culture that feels comfortable and authentic, you are creating a level of mutual respect.

This means when people have issues, whether they're at home, in the salon, or even with future employees, it doesn't matter if they still work for you or not. They trust you enough to leave their pride at the door.

Product Distribution

When you're working as a stylist and dreaming about owning a salon one day, you don't think about how you're going to sell and purchase your products. You think about being behind a chair, doing hair, and making money. But from experience, I know how important it is to get that selling process right, and as a *coach*, I know so many people are struggling with it.

Any salon owner can change or take on a product line at any time and become a distributor for that product if they want to. What I've found, though, is that new stylists are becoming overwhelmed, taking on line after line after line of new products without any capacity to sell them effectively.

To understand why we're in a place where product distribution has become the tough animal that it is, we have to step back and look at the trends.

Twenty years ago, if a distributor wanted to convert your salon to their product, they would have to meet and build a relationship with you. Often, this was the only way to get your hands on these products, so it was very much a game of negotiation. But these distributors would be experts on this product and train your stylists to become experts too. This meant that when your stylists sold the products to their clients, they knew exactly what they were talking about.

These days, this same market is unrecognizable.

If you want to purchase your products in person, you'll go to a beauty supply store or a little variety store on the corner that stocks what you want. You'll be lucky if there's more than one person working there or anyone with any knowledge of the product you are buying. They won't have any education on the products because their only job is to ring you up.

In reality, you don't even have to go out anymore to find your products. Most big brands will sell in bulk on Amazon. If you want to, you can supply your entire salon with a product you know nothing about.

The huge problem with this is that when you're a hairstylist, everybody needs to have education on the product in order to use the product. If you don't have that education, you're not going to use it correctly. If you're not using your products correctly, you're not going to be giving your clients a quality service.

You can't be successful if you're not educated on your products.

There is more than that going on, though. Because the competition is cheap, quick, and accessible, actual distributors are struggling to keep up. This means they've shifted their priorities from building relationships, exclusivity, and training with their clients to money-saving techniques.

We had an experience where we reached out to a distributor to help us with our products. They told us they would be with us in the salon, help us take orders, educate our stylists - give us the full one-on-one experience. However, after purchasing the entire line of products, we saw less and less of them. There was simply no follow-through.

The problem is that it's a high cost to the distributor to now offer all these things. Even when they have good intentions, they're simply not able to keep up with the demand.

What's more, the product companies (who can now sell on Amazon for very little expense) just keep reducing the markup that distributors can earn on their commission. It simply doesn't make sound business sense for a distributor to travel, build relationships, educate their client, and pay for shipping if they're only getting a 20% commission.

The only solution I've found as a salon owner who wants to become a distributor is to find a company that gives you a 100% markup. So if you buy it for $10, you're going to sell it for $20.

You will find, however, that the companies that give you that type of commission don't pay for advertising. So you have to consider the costs of doing your own advertising and legwork. It's a lot of work, but by building a relationship with the company and actually educating yourselves on the products you're using, you will earn the trust of your clients.

SECTION 4

Pain is NOT Beauty

Running a successful salon doesn't have to be painful. There are so many ways you can avoid mistakes, heartbreak and even running into money issues. I know from experience that the biggest quality a salon owner must have is resilience - and not everyone is up for the task. In this section, we're going to look at:

- The biggest mistakes you could make as a salon owner;
- How you change your headspace to envision success; and
- Changes you can make to create a salon your stylists believe in.

Chapter 5

So, You Want To Open A Salon?

> "Everything is always
> working out perfectly for me."

If you want to run your own successful commission salon, there are many ways you can go wrong, from your financial decisions, to who you're hiring, to the products you are using. But the first thing you have to do is take a long, hard look at yourself and ask the big question: "Am I cut out for this?"

Leading people is a gift and a skill that not everybody has. As a stylist, it's easy to fall into the trap of thinking that owning a salon is the next step in your career. But if you don't know how to run a business, I wouldn't recommend opening a salon.

But if you do, I want to explore some of the biggest mistakes you could make when you're just starting out.

The first thing you need to understand is how important it is to trust and listen to your gut. You will interact with so many people in this industry and, unfortunately, some of them will try to take advantage of you.

If you're approached by someone who's offering you the world, but your gut says something's off, it only takes a moment to do a bit of research to see if you're right. It might save you a lot of pain later down the road.

I was recently talking to a salon owner who told me that some people had approached them and offered to build their website. They would do the entire thing for this low price and give them a discount on any updates, partner with them to build their business, and network with them. They just gave them this entire story, so I asked them, "What's the catch?".

Here's the thing. As they say, "If it seems too good to be true, it probably is."

But as a new salon owner, you're so excited that somebody is promising you all these things that you don't realize that they're playing you until it's too late. It's not your fault when you're starting out because you're always feeling a bit desperate.

When I talked through this with the salon, we decided to trust the gut feeling and do a bit of research. We looked up the website and, you guessed it, the whole thing was a joke.

Now, these were good, sensible people who were going to give this man their money. It's even happened to me more times than I care to admit. I once had a woman reach out to me about doing my website. I thought I was being smart by calling up and checking all her references before I gave her half the money upfront. She took my money and never called me again.

So what I learned, after wasting so much money, is that sometimes you just have to build your own website. For someone who's not tech-savvy, that's pretty damn hard to do. But sometimes, if you're going to be successful, you have to have the resilience to figure it out.

There are so many things that are going to come up that you know nothing about when you own a business. You go in thinking you're just going to open the doors on a Monday morning, do some hair, and everything's going to be fine. But there's so much more to it. For example:

- Do you know how to market your business?
- Have you thought about your online presence (website, social media, etc.)?

- Do you have your state license?
- Have you created a handbook?
- Do you have payroll set up?
- Do you know how to do your employment taxes?
- Do you have an accountant?
- Have you talked to a financial advisor?

There are so many things that you don't think about or believe won't be needed when the reality is you will need all the help you can get.

You need to be able to go into this line of work knowing that you aren't going to get paid for at least five years, and the money you do spend on the business will be out of pocket. That situation takes a lot of financial preparation and restraint, especially because when you start, you will be working all day every day.

It is the most work you're ever going to do in your life. It's not going to be quick to get everything up and running. You have to want it that bad because there is nothing like the pressure of knowing you have 20 people whose families depend on *you*. You have to have the strongest work ethic because there will come the point when you simply cannot let those people down and give up. Also, if you're trying to create the tools you need to succeed while the business is already running, you may be losing some people.

Creating a whole business from scratch can be overwhelming without the support of the right people. It's the only shortcut you can take and still get things done right. That's why it is so important to get yourself a mentor or a coach. With Head Case coaching, we offer you these tools, so you don't have to spend sleepless nights creating a handbook or writing up policies like I did. It's the best way to equip yourself with the things you need to run your business successfully.

Money Issues

Coming back into the industry and opening a salon was such a huge decision. Partially it was difficult because I knew that balancing the books with work and looking after my family was about to get a hell of a lot harder. This is why I say, if you want to go into salon ownership as a stylist, you *have* to have a mind for business.

The first hurdle you face is financing. When I first started Head Case, I was told I was going to get an SBA loan (Small Business Administration loan). With reassurance from the vice president of the bank that the loan was going to come through, I signed the lease for my building and began work hiring my stylists. Then days went by, then weeks. I lost a couple of stylists just waiting for this money to land in my bank account.

Then the whole thing fell through.

I had 10 people ready to work and a five-year lease on my shoulders. I ended up opening it all up on credit cards. That hurt me for a long time, but I had to do it because so many people were depending on me.

My second huge hurdle was that my partner at the time was doing my books for me. He was also responsible for helping me get all the credit cards.

As that relationship deteriorated, it became a very messy situation. He was advising me to take on more loans and get myself into even more debt, and then I discovered that he had changed the log-ins for all of my accounts and money had moved so many times it was nearly impossible to follow.

When he finally left, I had no idea how to even start looking at our finances. No one had ever taught me how to create an LLC (Limited Liability Company) or sign up for QuickBooks™, or even access a business account.

It was a huge learning curve that I had to teach myself along the way. During that time, I did have a lot of setbacks and hurdles to overcome.
My main challenge was people trying to take advantage of me. You never learn how to handle that, and without the right mentors and support cultures around you, it's very easy to fall into that trap.

A lot of times, people would come into my salon and just assume I had all this money because of our surface-level success, even though I was barely making payroll.

By the time COVID hit, I was ready to quit. At that point, I was $100,000 in debt at a minimum. I still had a few years left on my lease and up to 20 employees to look after, who were now all isolating due to the pandemic.

The day we were told to close our doors and isolate, I went to the bank and got out a cashier's check for each of my employees, emptying out my checking account. I didn't know if we were going to open again or what was going to happen with the world. But I wanted to make sure that everyone was paid for the work they had done up until that moment so that they could take care of themselves.

I remember after I wrote the last check, I asked the woman at the bank how much money I had in my account, and she said $38. I was just so happy and so relieved it wasn't zero because it meant that everyone could get paid.

The sad thing was that the woman then said to me, "Do you know most people that came in before you emptied their bank account, and did not pay their staff?" Too many people put a lock on the door and cut off communication with their employees at that time. I couldn't believe it. When you have people who depend on you, you have a responsibility to them, even if it means you have to make sacrifices in your own life.

After that, I got a bunch of macaroni and cheese from Sam's Club (because that's all that was left after everyone had gone into a panic and cleaned it out) and got home to find that one of my employees decided to cash a check that he hadn't cashed yet. I finally went into the negative. When that happened, I said to myself, "I'm done. I'm so done."

I had no idea how to dig myself out of this hole, and the responsibility of looking after my team when I was surviving on mac and cheese was just too much.

Later, I remembered that a while back, I'd bought this online course with Dean Grazioso and Tony Robbins that I'd never had the chance to look at. It was lockdown, so I had nothing else to do. I started on these classes, and everything changed.

It started helping me change my mindset. I began to understand the control I had over this whole situation. I started getting my mental state right and not held down by all the anxiety. I started asking myself, "What am I going to do about it?"

I applied for another loan. It was meant to be my big brain wave that would save everyone. But it fell through *again*. I had to go back to a space where I could focus my mind and get my mental state right. I thought, "Okay, the loan didn't work. What am I going to do about it?"

When you're in those desperate times, you need that space to think clearly and make rational decisions. I broke down my situation with the help of people who actually knew what they were talking about, and I realized that the one thing I needed was a contact at a bank - a smaller bank than I had used before.

It turned out I already had one. My ex-husband's current wife worked at a local bank, so I called her and just asked the question, "Hey, do you know someone at the bank who can help me? I need to get a PPP loan." This is something they started offering to people during COVID to help businesses keep their workforce employed.

The president of the bank was on the phone with me an hour later, listening to my story. I told him that I had 20 employees who were relying on me and if I didn't get this loan I would have to shut down for good.

He just said, "No problem. I'll make sure you get it."

In total, we were closed for 51 days during the COVID pandemic, and the PPP loan saved the company.

Then our whole business just exploded when the fear of Covid died down. *Everyone* needed their hair done, and what's more, *everyone* wanted natural organic products. We were twice as busy as we had ever been, and every single member of my team stepped up. They worked their butts off and some offered to work seven days a week.

I paid off all of my debt within one year.

It became clear that the more I changed my mindset from anxiety and panic to focus on abundance, the more abundance I received. I spoke the affirmation to myself again and again:

"Everything is always working out perfectly for me."

Now What?

So, you've opened your salon, you've survived a pandemic, and money is starting to come in. Now what?

Some of the biggest hurdles I see that established salons trip over when they think they've become financially sustainable involve marketing. They get to a point where they think, "Well, we're doing great. Why should we bother anymore?" So they stop doing it or at least cut the budget to do other things.

But without marketing, you stop getting new clients. As soon as you stop getting new clients, your business will start to fail.

Years ago, there was a culture where people would be loyal and stay with their stylists through thick and thin. Even if they messed up their hair, clients would go back and get it changed by that same stylist.

You have to understand that this culture has shifted significantly. Thoughts in the industry currently are that seventy percent of first time clients, don't return to the same stylist or salon. It appears that that percentage is growing now. It's all because we now live in a world where inspiration and trends cycle so quickly that the old loyalty falls by the wayside. Most clients will be on platforms like Instagram every day, where they will see a new hairstyle or color they like. They might even see influencers or recommendations for different salons. It means that there has been this huge shift where people will explore and try a new stylist every single time they need (or want) their hair done.

This means you can't afford *not* to advertise because you simply don't keep the clients that you used to.

You have to set a budget aside for your marketing. There are a lot of inexpensive ways to promote and build your marketing presence yourself, but don't be afraid to outsource if you have access to reliable and talented support.

One of the simplest things you can do is set up a Google Business Profile. It's completely free and means that you can be officially listed on Google. It's a stamp of legitimacy that can reassure new clients, but it also helps naturally generate SEO (Search Engine Optimization) for your company. I highly recommend to update your page weekly with new photos and content for google to continue to recommend your salon.

By taking advantage of this and staying in the algorithm, we get at least 30,000 people that go to our profile every month. Without costing us a thing.

Once you start building these things, you have to keep them going. But it's also important to be aware that because you will continuously bring in new clients, you will need to make sure you have enough employees to look after them.

It's about properly looking at your production and being aware of how many stations you have, the days you are open, and if you have any chairs that aren't occupied on any of those days. If you have an empty chair, this is when I would start hiring. In fact, you should always be hiring.

Every stylist who comes to work with you will probably bring about five clients with them. Then each of those clients, if they enjoy the experience, will start bringing along their friends and family. This is how you grow your business.

Clients and stylists are people. People move, people leave, people die. It's just a fact you need to prepare for. But if you don't have a good culture, great customer service, or follow-through, then they're not going to stay with you anyway.

At Head Case, we have our books constantly booked for this very reason. But it's also because it's the only way to get quality stylists.

You can't hire every person who applies; you have to interview them extensively. Among the other obvious things, make sure that:

- They need to know about your salon and what it stands for;
- They have to have looked *you* up and researched who you are; and
- They have to give you a good enough reason why they want to be there.

After that first interview, they must be able to come in and do a practical. I don't care if they have been a salon professional for 30 years; you need to see what their skill level is before you hire them. For those who don't know what a "practical" is, it is when you have someone come into your salon and actually do a cut and color or hair color or whatever you want them to do to show you their level of competence.

Some people won't like this. There's this assumption in this industry that people who have been working in it longer have stronger skills, but this simply isn't true.

Often people become complacent with their education and don't push themselves to work harder and improve.

On the other hand, if someone is willing to humble themselves for a practical, it puts them in good stead with the rest of the team. It also allows you to:

- Give existing stylists the opportunity to watch, interact with them, and offer their opinions;
- Get a much stronger idea of how they interact with other people and how they treat the client;
- Get an insight into how comfortable they are asking questions; and
- See how they take *feedback*.

It's a tryout so that you can find the right people that will complement and grow a loving culture.

Too many people will hire someone just because they have a license. It might be a cheaper process to do this, but you just don't know how much it will cost you in the long term if that person clashes with your values as an organization.

This leads me to the final mistake I see established salons dealing with: not preparing themselves for heartbreak.

There will always come a time when you have an employee, whom you love and trust, who will move on. Even when you truly believe that they're in it with you until the end, it still hurts even when they leave on good terms, and you can wish them well.

But when things get complicated, and people lie about you or steal clients, it can be a real challenge to overcome emotionally.

What you have to do is reframe your thinking about it: the fact that they left is actually a blessing.

The reason why people leave is that they're not sold on your business, and people pick up on that energy. If someone is causing a rift in your business, maybe even talking badly about you, it is so much better if that person steps away.

It is the perfect opportunity for a fresh start and for you to open your heart to someone new.

How You Fix It

Your team culture is your number one priority because if you don't have your healthy team culture, then you're going to keep losing your stylists.

Every day while I'm driving or doing my hair, I'm listening to talks and podcasts on growing my mindset and my business. I know that, as a salon owner, you have to always be spinning your plates.

- Focus on the health of your team, mentally and physically;
- Develop your team culture, do team building together outside of the salon; and
- Expand yourself so that you're always able to take care of your staff.

If you're not in the right mindset every single day, then it will lead to failure. Everything you think, say, and do is going to ripple through your entire business. When I'm struggling with my emotions, I know that I need a safe space to let them out.

What helps me immediately is meditation. I focus on the problem - not as something negative, but as something we can find benefits in. I then identify the immediate solutions so that we can tackle the issue in a practical way. When I'm finished, and I've been through this process, I can then walk out onto the salon floor without needing to air any dirty laundry.

I tell this to my coaching clients all the time: if you're depressed, you will lose your salon. You need to be able to surround yourself with people who will build you up and support your business when you stumble. This is why I highly recommend hiring a coach who knows what you're going through and can give you the confidence you need to take the next steps.

As we already know, it's not just your mental health that you need to take care of. The physical well-being of both yourself and your stylists is so important.

If you want to learn about how you can transition your salon to be green, organic, and sustainable, we are starting a new yearly conference called the 'Sustainable Salon Summit.' See www.sustainablesalonsummit.com During the summit, we will be hearing from organizations that will help you expand and grow in ways you may never have even thought about before. Key speakers will share business tips from financial, marketing, to leadership. A few of our partners include:

- **Green Circle Salons** - a company that can recycle all of your waste (including hair) to reduce landfill, methane levels and protect our planet.
- **PHOREST** - a software system that can track everything you need to market and build your clientele sustainably.
- **Vish** - a color-safe system that measures hair color products down to the gram. That means zero unnecessary waste, and it saves you money. Best thing to happen to a salon owner!
- **NATULIQUE™** - our Danish partners in distributing organic, sustainable products with over 20 years of experience in the industry.
- **Sustain Beauty Co** - founders of eco heads and sustainable salon tool distribution.

Each one of these companies is focused on how they're impacting the planet at the same time as they are making products or creating solutions. Sustainable is a lot more than just recycling or using chemical-free products; it's an entire ecosystem of business.

SECTION 5

Community Over Competition

The beauty industry can be a place that just breeds competition. Don't get me wrong, I'm here for a little competition, but I am passionate about creating salon communities that care for each other *more* than winning as an individual. In this section, I'm going to talk about:

- How to build a supportive and loving environment in your salon;
- What it is that truly motivates us and makes us want to succeed; and
- What this sustainable model of business could look like in the future.

Chapter 6

Building The Tribe

> "Surround yourself with people
> who will have your back
> at the end of the day."

When it comes down to it, success for me looks like a loving salon culture. When people join my team at the very beginning, they are told that they are no longer working as individuals; they work as a *team* to serve a greater purpose. We support each other and grow together as artists and as people.

Without competition, we are able to work as a unit. If someone calls up a stylist asking for a bob, they might say, "I actually know another stylist here who does amazing bobs," and share their client with someone else.

Everyone who walks through our doors is a Head Case client, not an individual client. Everyone will greet them and work together to make sure they have the best possible experience. Making sure people aren't left on their own or without a beverage in their hand or without a compliment or two. If stylists are rushed off their feet, someone else will step in to help them finish sweeping up hair or grab a coffee for them. Everyone goes so above and beyond in their kindness.

I'm so lucky to have the team that I have. We've spent so much time building and investing, and loving each other to create this team as the tribe that it is today.

There are always highs and lows on the salon floor, but sometimes it's okay to break down some of the formalities of work and organize events to do together. I have the team over to my house for dinner and karaoke or we hit the local bowling joint so we can all have a night off and have fun. Everyone actually gets to be themselves.

It's so important to build this kind of rapport and team camaraderie. Another one of the things I love to do is close down the salon a few hours early and throw the stylists a little hair care party.

We're always so busy, so sometimes this might be the only chance for our stylists to sit down, relax and get their hair done. No one wants to go home after a whole day of working on other people's hair to give themselves a balayage that takes three hours, but if you have a team of four people working on it (and a glass of champagne), you'll get it done in no time.

These parties build up everyone's self-esteem, especially for the stylists, because they're looking good and they're feeling good. It creates a beautiful culture inside the salon.

Another part of a community is between salon owners. We have been competitive for too long, and it is time to come together for support. Who better to understand us than our peers? I learn so much from fellow salon owners and distributors that have been imperative to my growth as a person and a salon owner. Join our community of incredible salon owners by visiting www.headcasecoaching.com.

Love Each Other

At Head Case, we have one golden rule: we do not tolerate negativity or gossip. There is always so much of it in this industry and it can make or break your business. From the beginning of their contracts, my stylists know what our expectations are and that breaking this rule could result in the termination of their employment.

Then if they still do it, we always pull them aside to have a conversation. I always want to get deep about it, so I ask them how they are or if there's anything going on at home. Basically, to try and get to the root of the issue and try and work out a solution.

If you're being negative for the sake of being negative, then I have no time for you. But, the beauty industry is so different from any other industry in the sense that everything is just so much more personal. You can't simply fire a person on a whim, because even though they're acting up, they could still be a good stylist that the clients and the team absolutely love.

That interconnection is why it's so important to go deeper. What they are struggling with could be their own issues, their own pain or something external that is making them start to mess up or be a problem. If you can get to that inner pain and help them from there, on a personal level, suddenly the difficulties they're having at work start to improve.

The key is gratitude. I've given every single one of my employees when they start a book on gratitude called "The Magic" by Rhonda Byrne. If someone ever starts complaining, I'll always ask, "Did you do your gratitude this morning?"

Part of creating a successful and loving culture in a salon is finding a cause that everyone can get behind and support. It unites us all in ways you wouldn't think about and helps establish a sense of achievement beyond the day to day client work.

At Head Case we are passionate about cruelty-free products, and even more, we just love our animals. So, we started doing this big fundraiser every year where our clients can get a free blowout - as long as they bring a 25lb bag of dog food for us to donate to the Humane Society.

Everyone gets so excited about it because it's very important to everybody that we support this charity. No one gets any money out of it, but we always end up donating about 1,800 lb of dog food.

Organic Success

For some time now, I've been building a coaching program with my team, and it's so funny how many times I'll suggest something that Angela doesn't agree with or doesn't think will work. What's even funnier is all the times she'll come back to me a few weeks later and say, "Oh my God, you're absolutely right." Nobody is doing what we're doing, but more importantly, it actually *works.*

For instance, most salons will implement a 'level' structure with their stylists. A level 1 stylist is usually younger with less experience in the field - however, they meet the skill level set by the salon. Whereas a level 4 stylist is usually in a more senior role. They will typically have a lot of experience in all areas of work and have spent time learning and developing their skill set. As you would expect, the higher your level, the higher amount of commission you can earn.

This hierarchy model that so many salons use is based on the maturation of a skill set that may or may not have been further developed over the years. I used this system in my corporate salon and I felt it created a more competitive than cohesive team.

For so long, the industry has been teaching and doing the same things over and over. We know that it isn't a sustainable way to be successful in this industry, especially right now with the new 'Gen Z' generation coming in. They want equality and innovation - whereas your veteran stylists who have been working for 20 years want recognition and higher pay.

The truth is, it doesn't matter if you've been working for 20 years; if someone else is working twice as hard and getting better results, they should be paid fairly for their work. Your performance and how you treat your clients should be the only thing you consider when you look at the numbers. If stylists want to get paid more, they have to step up.

At Head Case, every single one of our stylists has the same opportunity and is treated the same. They can make as much money as they want. It all depends on performance. That is how our commission system works at Head Case. A lot of people don't understand it, but it helps everybody be on an equal playing field.

Another thing we changed was the way in which we sell our products. It's something that so many stylists struggle with because they're not trained in sales, and they often feel uncomfortable pitching to their clients.

We tried so many things to increase our sales numbers and encourage them to grow their confidence:

- **Confrontation -** Brandy and I would bring them in to ask them why they were not meeting the goal, set new expectations, and then meet with them two weeks later. Each time was the same result. But constantly telling your stylists that they aren't performing to a high enough standard can kill their motivation. It just generates guilt and creates a negative culture in your salon.

- **Training** - We held so many training sessions to try and boost the confidence of our stylists. I even gave them a consultation form that went step-by-step through how they could make a sale. This wasn't effective because stylists are *artists,* not salespeople; it's not who they are.

- **Financial incentive** - We increased the commission on any retail products by 10% every time a stylist exceeded their sales goal. But we quickly realized that money wasn't a big enough motivator.

The problem with all of these methods is that people respond to different forms of motivation for different reasons. In order to achieve organic growth in your sales, you need to understand your team, and what it is that inspires them.

For instance, some of our team responded really well to the training we did, whereas others didn't step up until the financial incentive was introduced. Even then, we had people who struggled to hit their targets.

The way around this is to break it down even further and understand what it is your stylists actually need in order to *want* to reach these goals.

For many, saying you'll get a 10% or a 20% increase in sales commission doesn't sound like a lot. However, reframing that into a tangible number by saying instead, "You could be earning an additional $700 every week if you do this," you might suddenly have a lot more interest. You should know your stylists and if they're saving up for a car, maybe, or in desperate need of a vacation. That kind of extra money could be a huge incentive for them.

You could go further still by celebrating the people who do meet their sales targets. Perhaps even presenting them their paychecks in front of the rest of the team so that everyone else can see what they're missing out on. But money isn't always a motivator for some people. At

Head Case, I discovered that a lot of stylists really value their service commission.

Because we don't use the level system, everyone starts on an equal playing field when it comes to their commission. If they have a high commission, it's because they've worked hard and they've earned it. Our stylists take pride in it because it is a measurement of their identity, of how well they're doing as beauticians.

We implemented a rule that if a stylist didn't sell a minimum of $150 dollars of product a week - a very low target - we would drop their service commission to offset the loss in revenue.

Honestly? I wasn't very popular that week. But what happened was that everyone started to really support and help each other because they wanted everyone to succeed. Nobody wanted to lose their service commission, even if they were still afraid of selling retail. But now they were in control and the pressure was off.

Discovering what truly motivates your employees is vital to creating a sustainable workplace. It's been an amazing thing for me to witness - going on this journey, looking into every way, shape, or form we could to solve this issue in order to help them get to that point.

Suddenly, those talks in the back office turned into the stylists excitedly telling me how many sales they closed that day. Their sales assessments came along in leaps and bounds. As a company, we started to see a huge increase in our retail profit.

But most importantly, we grew as a team and created a culture that loved and supported one another.

Family Matters

It's so important when you are building your business to surround yourself with people that you trust and with family if you can. These are always going to be the people who will have your back at the end of the day.

I'm so lucky that I am able to share my business with my daughter. There is no one else I would rather work with, and she has the best talent for leadership that I have ever seen.

But that's not to say there haven't been some challenges. My daughter and I have had our differences and 'big old fights' both publicly and privately. There are many things I wish we could have done differently, especially the way we handled some of our issues and where we aired the dirty laundry.

We fought a lot in the beginning, and to be honest with you, it was so bad we lost a few people. It's always complex when you have a personal family history that overlaps with your professional life. Keeping those two things from clashing is a skill that we are still working on to this day, but. But through it all, there was always underlying love and respect. We're so much better now.

Even though she'd never give me a compliment to my face to save her life, I once heard her say to someone, "My mom's the hardest working person I know. She just loves everyone, no matter what."

I know it's probably not easy trying to make your own way in the world with your mom at the helm. I'm so grateful to her for putting up with me and allowing me to watch her grow into this amazing leader.

It was a journey for me, too; we've learned so much from each other. I also had to learn to loosen the reins and let her learn things on her own. There's so much that failure can teach her that I could never be able to put into words. But hell, keeping your mouth shut when you know it's going to happen is hard. You have to know when to back off and let the other person make the decisions. Then stand by them, whatever the outcome.

But the word 'family' at Head Case goes much deeper than just blood. My team is also my chosen family.
Don't get me wrong, sometimes you want to kill them, and sometimes they drive you crazy. But that is what family does. At the end of the day, you still love them no matter what.

If there is something going on, you try to fix it. You find out what the reason is, and you say, "How can I help you?"

We do that because with family comes the expectation that someone will always be there for you. If you're having an off day, we will notice. We will help you get back on track with your clients or grab you a change of clothes or whatever it is they might need but do not know to ask.

But in return, you have to talk to us and 99% of the time, if you ask someone if they're okay, they will say they are fine. Your "co-worker" won't push it. Your "family" will push it. At the end of the day, they will know you better than anyone else and know when you're off and need to talk to somebody.

Brandy, my daughter, is so good at this; she knows how to get to the point. She'll just tell you, "Are you going to talk to me about this or my mom?" She knows instinctively when people are trying to bury their issues instead of letting them out.

If everyone on the team has high standards, they will hold everyone else to the same standard. When you, as the salon owner, put your stylists before your clients, you are showing your stylists that standard.

Chapter 7

The Voice Of Sustainability

> "This is just the beginning."

Stepping into the person that I want to be, the voice of sustainability for an industry that is hurting so many people, is definitely going to be an ongoing process. I have learned so much over my years of experience as a manager and a salon owner. But every day, I'm challenging myself to seek out further information about what is out there.

If you get nothing else from this book, I want to empower you right now to do the research you need to make the right decisions for yourself and your family. Whether it's for your kids or for your chosen family, we all deserve to live happy, healthy, *beautiful* lives.

Salons across the country are filled with so many wonderful people who deserve to know how to run their businesses sustainably. They deserve to know the truth about the chemicals they are using and how to transition their salons to greener products. They deserve to know how to build up their own businesses and make a 6-figure profit. They deserve to be loved by the people around them in a culture that supports them without hesitation.

I gravitated to this industry because the salon was always my comfort place, and that kind of peace gets in your blood. You can't just shake it off. I know this is true of so many other people too.

Often, people like this are those who are already struggling with their own problems. They may be people who are seeking out a place they can be accepted and loved when they might not have any other option.

These are the people who listen and touch, and care for you every day of their lives. They deserve so much more respect than they often receive, and yet they still keep doing what they do.

The reason I started my pro-coaching service was to help my clients in all areas of their life, not just as salon owners and stylists. What I offer is my wisdom, my truth, and my complete respect for what you do and how you do it. I want to help you grow your business, your clients, your stylists, AND yourself.

Together we can:

- Help you gain confidence in the conversations you have with your clients and stand your ground with your decisions;
- Find clients that can't get enough of what *you* have to offer;
- Guarantee your clients keep coming back;
- Protect your energy by regulating your mindset;
- Make more money and relieve the pressure of making payroll;
- Develop a plan for your future;
- Help you understand who you are and where you want to be; and, finally,
- Take that journey to feeling truly happy with yourself and the life *you* have created.

We also offer two different certifications. The first is our "sustainability" certification after completing our sustainable salon business course. You will be giving beauty waste a new life and joining the fight against climate change.

The second is a coaching certification. If you finish our coaching sessions and feel passionate about developing your own coaching skills, we offer 1-1 and group coaching training for any salon owner or stylist.

I strongly believe that there could be an amazing opportunity within the beauty industry to develop new ways of "coaching."

If you think about how many of our clients sit in our chairs and tell us about their lives and their troubles but won't go to see a therapist - I think there is a huge need to train up our stylists.

As a successful stylist, you are naturally intuitive to people's emotions. Every day, you are working with people without having the core skill set to properly handle their emotional well-being. Often this can lead to discomfort or the stylist taking on the client's emotional energy, and it can start to have a negative impact on the stylist's own well-being.

If we start training stylists as coaches, we could make a huge impact in all areas of our client's lives, not just their hair. If we equip our teams with the tools to notice when our clients need more support or maybe even seem suicidal, they can learn to talk to them more appropriately and get them the help they need.

As a coach and a salon owner, I want to keep thinking creatively about all the ways we can change this industry. Sometimes the only way to identify a problem is to see it for yourself, which is why I also offer hands-on, in-person support to salons that really need to shake things up.

If you're not based in Texas or prefer online resources, I also offer a free online consultation program to help identify which areas of your life and business you need help with the most. Our methods are cutting-edge and innovative and designed for salon professionals, business owners, and management. Find out more at www.headcasecoaching.com

Our Future

Creating a sustainable beauty industry starts with you reading this book. It starts with the changes you make to your own salons and spending habits. It starts with all the clients you talk to and all the people they share that conversation with.

But this is just the beginning.

There are so many people out there who don't know and don't *want* to know about this crisis. Sometimes it is easier to bury your head in the sand and stick to your creature comforts than to step out and do something different. I don't blame them. Going against the grain is hard and sometimes even terrifying. But the only way to ensure lasting, positive change is to lead by example.

I've tried speaking in beauty schools about sustainability, but it became very apparent that they weren't ready for that information. It's frustrating when some institutions don't care enough about their students to give them the tools they really need to succeed. I have to believe there will be more opportunities to get this information into curriculums. It's the only way these kids are going to come out of school with an education that will have a positive impact on our industry.

I want to use my voice to give hope that we can change. I want to reach not just the ten or twenty people in my salon, not just *you,* but everyone. There are 35,866 active salon licenses in just Texas alone and almost a million across the country. So, we've got a lot of ground to cover.

I will be sending a copy of this book to the environmental offices of the government in each state, along with a proposal to meet with them and an offer to work with them as a consultant on this issue.

Those that respond will be highlighted on my website.

Testimonials

Employee Reviews

"Working at Head-case is definitely one of the most wonderful experiences in my journey as an artist.

 The culture in the studio is a constant strive for that of care, transparency, and family as a team.
Introducing organic products to the studio has been life-changing to many of our guests and me. As a hairdresser, I can say that I have experienced an absolute difference from working with non-harsh chemicals versus other products out there in the industry. They are pleasant to work with while giving me peace of mind for the health of my guest, myself, and the health of my peers."

Rissa Alvarado

"Working at Head Case Hair Studio has quite literally changed my life. The culture is unlike any place I have ever worked. These stylists and owners are extremely talented and breed positivity and teamwork.

I have never felt more like I belong somewhere than I do here. The bonus is being able to fully stand behind the product we use. I have seen Natulique truly change not only my hair, but countless clients in the year that I have been here. **I have finally found my forever salon, and I could not be happier"**

Heather Charland

"Have you ever walked into a salon and just knew you belonged there? I did. The first time I walked into HeadCase, I knew I belonged. As a seasoned stylist of 21 years, it can sometimes be a challenge to find a home that embraces all that you bring. I have worked with all the harsh chemicals of this industry and even some very well-known natural brands that are not so natural.

Head Case has done the research and provides only the best and most natural product for us to use behind the chair. They care about their staff and clients, from the products we use to the way we recycle to protect our planet. I love talking with clients seeking a like-minded salon to bring health to their hair and life. I can't wait to see where Head Case takes us."

Erika Wightman

"I have known Kelley for over 13 years, and in that time, I have seen her go from the store manager to the proud owner of the first hair salon in the area to offer clean, sustainable beauty that performs at a high standard. It wasn't something that came easy.

I saw Kelley go through a hard-working journey and a journey that changed many lives, including mine.

I've worked with many haircare lines and for different salons, but working at Head Case for Kelley has been different. I was just a number at other salons, but I feel cared for here.

Kelley has found the cleanest professional haircare line to ensure her employees' health is not at risk, as well as our clients. Kelley is invested in offering only the best and truly cares for her staff and the community. I am very thankful to work for her and look forward to going to work knowing Kelley always has my back.

I know we will keep thriving because, at the core of it all, Kelley's belief that EVERYONE deserves access to clean beauty started this whole journey, and it keeps being the drive to raise the industry's standards so that it becomes the only option.

Myrna Velez

"Working at Head Case is and has been such a great experience! Everyone is family to me, and I couldn't have asked for a better one.

From starting out as an apprentice to a FULLY BOOKED stylist, the amount of fantastic support to expanding my career into a Barber Stylist is amazing!

Anytime I wanted more education and support in my craft, they offered it and supported me and my development as an individual in the business and as an artist.

They have pushed me to be the best I can be and still are to this day. Head Case makes sure I grow, and having this team supporting me is a great experience! No one is competing with each other. We all help each other like an ecosystem that works together for a common goal.

The work environment is so positive! We have such a blast, even on super stressful weekend-packed days. The managers always have your back and best interests in mind in every situation; you can go to them for anything.

I have really found my work home. I'm not going anywhere; I'm so excited for the future of this salon and so very thankful to be a part of it."

Veronica Nalepka

"I love working for Head Case because working with organic products helps me stay healthy and makes me feel comfortable using products that don't damage the hair. The bonus is that everyone is friendly."

Jose Lopez

"I love working at Head Case because we protect our hair health, bodies, and environment. I love that we use clean, cruelty-free, and organic products that provide even better results for different hair goals but in a safer, cleaner way. **We have a caring team with the end goal of doing better for ourselves, our clients, and each other."**

Jessica Dinh

Salon Owner Reviews

"As a new salon owner, trying to figure everything out can be scary. Wanting to get everything right the first time is stressful. That's why I am incredibly grateful for Kelley and her amazing team. Being able to COUNT ON someone is rare these days. They helped in countless ways guide me through the process. **A true hands-on team that is there for you when you need them. Kelley and her team have so much experience and knowledge to really help take my business to the next level! They have helped give me the tools and knowledge to feel confident in running my business.** They have worked tirelessly and enthusiastically to help me on this journey. **I couldn't have done it without them and their support. If you want to feel unequivocally supported and get the business training you need, I highly recommend them!**"

Jennifer Finkelstein

"About a year ago, I was looking for a better product to bring to my growing salon. I was unhappy and underwhelmed by my current product line. After being introduced to Kelley at Innovative Beauty, I knew I had found the perfect team. Not only has Natulique changed my life, but it's also changed my clients.

We love the chemical-free processing that gives us better results than I could've imagined. Being a new salon owner has had its share of obstacles, but with kelley in my corner, I know there is nothing she can't help me with. **If you're looking to transform your salon or business, Kelley and her team are where you need to start."**

Ashley Taylor

"I recently opened my studio using Natulique exclusively. After 15 years with the same company, I say this was a huge career change for me. I could not be happier with my transition. **I have had so much support from the crew at Innovative Beauty Distributors. They made sure to get me all available training materials and education.** Kelley even invited me to the Head Case Salon to observe! Ordering is very simple, and deliveries are quick. There are great rewards for purchases. The crew has also helped me troubleshoot some color formulas.

If your clients are not happy, no one is happy. I have a clientele that has been brand loyal over the course of my career and some even before that—hard converts. I can tell you they are happy! They are purchasing retail! They are coming back! They are telling their friends and family! We have better gray coverage than with the previous color line. **The hair looks and feels more luxurious. My clients and I have a clean conscience knowing we can look and feel amazing with no compromise. Sustainable beauty is the future. Non-negotiable!"**

Laura Zen

Next Steps

Join Kelley's Head Case Coaching:

You can benefit by joining my Head Case Coaching. For more information, visit www.HeadCaseCoaching.com .

Visit Head Case Salon:

Kelley's salon, Head Case, is located at 1200 Keller Parkway, Suite 400, Keller TX 76248. For appointments go to www.HeadCaseHairStudio.com
or call 1(682) 593-7425.

Try NATULIQUE™ For Yourself!

You can get Kelley's certified organic products from Innovative Beauty Distributors, right next door at Suite 300. Another option is to order online at www.NatuliqueTX.com or 1(817) 916-8899.

Find out more about our annual Sustainable Summit. Speakers include Sophia Hilton, Green Circle Salons, PHOREST, Vish and NATULIQUE™ .

About the Author

Kelley Swing, the Millionaire Voice of Sustainable Beauty, lives in Keller, Texas with her husband, Gregory and their animal family (two dogs and a cat).

She is a certified business coach through Mindvalley Evercoach. When not in her salon or helping other salons to become Million Dollar Sustainable Salons, she continues her own education to keep abreast of the latest trends, studies and options for a more sustainable world.

Kelley is an expert beauty industry advisor to the Rolling Stones Culture Counsel. She has published numerous articles on their site:

https://council.rollingstone.com/u/9be
cd93a-96be-49d2-99d7-bdb009a91a33

Kelley loves to spend time playing with her grandchildren.